ALZHEIMER'S IS
INEXORABLE

ALZHEIMER'S IS INEXORABLE

True Grit and Fortitude needed

Brian Scott Edwards, MD, FNLA

Library of Congress Control Number: 2021925434
ISBN: Hardcover   978-1-6698-0492-5
                   Softcover   978-1-6698-0491-8
                   eBook   978-1-6698-0490-1

Print information available on the last page.

Rev. date: 12/23/2021

To order additional copies of this book, contact:
Xlibris
844-714-8691
www.Xlibris.com
Orders@Xlibris.com
836829

A question in your nerves is lit
Yet you know there is no answer fit
To satisfy, ensure you not to quit
To keep it in your mind and not forget
That it is not he, or she, or them, or it
That you belong to.
—Bob Dylan, "It's Alright, Ma
(I'm Only Bleeding)"

From Internet Applied Psychology

Five Characteristics of Grit

1. Courage
2. Conscientiousness: being thorough, careful or vigilant
3. Perseverance
4. Passion

The courage we all have to find within ourselves day after
day typically is not physical courage, but the moral courage to
remain true to all other virtues and to persevere in the face of
adversity. In this sense courage is the conscious act of free will.
—Stephen Grimble, *For Love & Liberty*, p. 272

CONTENTS

Foreword ix

Introduction xi

Chapter 1   Merry Christmas 1
Chapter 2   Happy Birthday 2
Chapter 3   Resolution? 3
Chapter 4   Michael J. Fox 4
Chapter 5   Irony of All Ironies 8
Chapter 6   Living dangerously...10
Chapter 7   How Can I Measure if My Alzheimer's Is
            Getting Worse? 11
Chapter 8   Alpha-Lipoic Acid 13
Chapter 9   Predicting How Many Good Years I Will Have 16
Chapter 10 Annual Visit to Florida Neurologist 19
Chapter 11 Trip to Boston to Visit Grandsons...........................21
Chapter 12 Choline..24
Chapter 13 Update on Fish Oil Levels.................................26
Chapter 14 Courage 28
Chapter 15 Return to Kansas 30
Chapter 16 Cleaning the Brain of Its Toxins? 31
Chapter 17 *A Tattoo on My Brain* Review: Part I 32
Chapter 18 *A Tattoo on My Brain* Review: Part II.....................35
Chapter 19 *A Tattoo on My Brain* Review: Part III 36
Chapter 20 The Smell of Baking Bread 37
Chapter 21 *A Tattoo on My Brain* Review: Part IV 39
Chapter 22 *A Tattoo on My Brain* Review: Part V....................41
Chapter 23 *A Tattoo on My Brain* Review: Part VI....................42
Chapter 24 Diets for Early Alzheimer's.................................. 44

Chapter 25 Amazon Review of *A Tattoo on My Brain*.....................46
Chapter 26 Update on a New AZ Drug...47
Chapter 27 Memory Is Not What It's Cracked Out to Be..............50
Chapter 28 National Weight Control Registry Survey....................51
Chapter 29 Life Goes On Even with Alzheimer's...........................53
Chapter 30 Minor Staircase Disaster..58
Chapter 31 Executive Function Challenge....................................59
Chapter 32 I Enjoy My Mornings...60
Chapter 33 Takeaways from Bredesen's Podcast on Fasting...........62
Chapter 34 Climbing the Bredesen ReCODE Supplement Ladder... 64
Chapter 35 A New Fun Experience with My Wife.........................67
Chapter 36 The Cheapest and Easiest Way to Try to Prevent
            Progression of Alzheimer's...70
Chapter 37 Cognitive Reserve with Alzheimer's............................74
Chapter 38 Fourth MRI For a Nontreatment Trial.......................75
Chapter 39 *On Pluto*: First Review..77
Chapter 40 *On Pluto*: Second Review..80
Chapter 41 *On Pluto*: Third Review...83
Chapter 42 Let Me Finish My Damn Sentence!............................86
Chapter 43 Review of *The First Survivors of Alzheimer's* by
            Dr. Dale Bredesen..87
Chapter 44 Supplements Advised by Isaacson and Chris Ochner...89
Chapter 45 Return from Three Weeks in Paris During
            COVID-19...90
Chapter 46 Final Advice for Everyone..93
Chapter 47 Decision to End Long Driving Trips...........................96

Final Word...101

FOREWORD

I am honored to be asked by Brian to write the FOREWORD to his fourth book on his journey with Alzheimer's. He and I have been friends for over fifty years. Brian grew up with two older brothers. His oldest brother Donald and I worked together in a clinical laboratory at Kings County Hospital in Brooklyn NY for a number of years. His middle brother, Steve, was the same age as me and we met at a YMCA church league softball game and realized we lived close to each other. So, we became very close friends for many years. I was frequently at the Edward's home growing up and Brian, Steve and I grew up playing basketball every winter at the church league during our Jr and Sr High School years. We've remained friends throughout the years watching each other's children grow up.

I remember the day Brian told us he had Alzheimer's disease in March 2018. We were in Maui on vacation with childhood friends. Of course, we were very surprised and talked about it for quite a while. He had a diagnosis of early onset disease but that did not stop him from tackling it with the same determination he tackled college, medical school, residencies, and board certifications in two medical specialties. Most people do not want to be informed of a diagnosis where they feel there is little or no hope. Brian is not that way; he keeps current with the latest research and treatments. As a physician, Brian is very health conscientious and clearly wants to teach others by writing books based on his experiences and his advice. Brian covers lots of interesting topics in this book including medication advice for those with diabetes mellitus, weight loss and prevention of heart disease and stroke. Clearly Brian has kept up to date with his knowledge of these areas including the latest meds and supplements to use.

Brian will continue to live his life with great interest in travel and learning about living with Alzheimer's; and also teaching us who are lucky enough to read his books and continue to be his friend.

Chris Bentsen
Gig Harbor, WA

INTRODUCTION

Personal History

When I first thought of the title "Alzheimer's Is Inexorable," I thought it would be appropriate for *year 4*, as I expected to really decline this year in 2021. Now I am not so certain. I still believe Alzheimer's is inexorable, as there is no cure and none on the horizon.

I have done well in the last three years, beyond my expectations. (Year 5 title: "Doing Better than Expected with Alzheimer's," subtitle: "Trying Not to Fall Off a Cliff")

In my first three books, I told people to avoid the false hope of nostrums. I wrote critiques on *The End of Alzheimer's Program*. However, with Dr. Dale Bredensen's second book, titled *The End of Alzheimer's Program*, I read about the continued success of Julie Gilbert, who was homozygous for Alzheimer's with E4/E4, family history, and what seemed to be early-onset dementia at age forty-six.

Now seven years later, she helped write the Program book.

With the advent of COVID-19, I had the time to do a year-long program of ReCODE designed by Dr. Dale Bredensen. To support this optimistic outlook was the discovery of the work of Dr. Isaacson at Cornell. He has a similar philosophy and also has had some success treating early-onset Alzheimer's with a patient named Lauren Miller Rogen.

Now that there are papers published reporting these successes, I am hopeful my prognosis to stay in mild cognitive impairment is much better for a much longer time than two years, which is achieved with the medication Namzaric alone.

Thus in 2021, as I enter the Bredensen ReCODE protocol with the Atma Clinic in Lawrence, Kansas, I will look at a program of nostrums in the hope of maintaining my mental status quo.

CHAPTER 1

Merry Christmas
December 25, 2020

I am watching *The Christmas Chronicles 2*. This might be one of those times it's good to have Alzheimer's.

I love Kurt Russell and Goldie Hawn. I thought I would watch this movie and turn it off for being so silly. I have to say I love it. It makes me feel so good.

CHAPTER 2

Happy Birthday
December 28, 2020

Despite the title of this book, I am very optimistic about next year. Three years after my diagnosis of Alzheimer's was made, I am delighted with my present mental state.

I am hoping to reach my seventieth birthday next December 2021. I hope to spend it with my three grandsons and put that photo of us together in my book. After my wife and I get vaccinated for COVID-19, we plan to take a great trip in Europe.

CHAPTER 3

Resolution?
January 2, 2021

I gave up on doing New Year's resolutions a long time ago. I resolve to lose weight every day. Once I get the COVID-19 vaccine, I plan to get back to the gym to do more weight lifting. I have done well in 2020 with walking ten thousand steps a day and doing curls, triceps reverse curls, and overhead presses with five-pound weights. I try to do twenty to thirty slow repetitions in each set. The tone in my biceps is much improved.

CHAPTER 4

Michael J. Fox

January 8, 2021

Michael J. Fox is a profile in grit in dealing with a horrendous disease, Parkinson's disease. In his third book on his PD titled *No Time Like the Present*, he writes, "I will go through any amount of pain or pressure to achieve my goal."

I remember thinking I saw Mr. Fox at the MCI airport in Kansas City. I knew the hospital I was doing an Infectious Disease Fellowship had an excellent Parkinson's department. I knew of his diagnosis of Parkinson's disease. He was with a much taller blond woman. I caught Michael's eye as I passed him, and we nodded to each other. He did not seem disabled.

Since then I have loved seeing him on TV. *The Good Wife* and the Fireman series. He clearly showed his disability in those episodes. He writes about these roles in his third autobiography, *No Time Like the Future*.

An optimist looks at his future.

His books are autobiographical about his trials and tribulations since being diagnosed with Parkinson's disease in 1991.

I have not read the previous best-selling memoirs. I recently purchased this new third book because it struck me how he used his personal experiences with Parkinson's to write the book. I have not been able to find another first person narrative such as myself with Alzheimer's to document the experience in a diary format.

Early into the book, I envied his excellent humor and excellent writing ability. He writes about his character, Louis Canning, in *The Good Wife* on page 32. "I know from experience that people have an aversion to anyone who moves differently."

"Louis Canning succeeded in preempting that reaction by projecting a friendly and forthcoming demeanor."

People are surprised I have come public with my diagnosis. I think it is similar to the stigma of cancer. I want to reinforce the idea that Michael presents on his "philosophy of less is more" on page 33. Despite his decreased motor abilities, he has found "there is more to less than I thought." I want to decrease the stigma of having Alzheimer's. I am not ashamed of my diagnosis. After three years and one month, I show that memory is not all it is cracked out to be. I think Michael's movement obstacles would be much more difficult for me to deal with.

Michael says on page 65, "More difficult and difficult to accept is the diminishment of movement ... it's a lesson in humility." For me, there is no shame and few obstacles to a great life other than returning to work. Learning to control my anger is a challenge.

In many ways, I envy aspects of Mike's life and his personality and his courage and determination to learn to play golf. I gave up golf after too many golf balls lost in the lake. His coterie of famous stars that support his efforts are examples. Still I would not change places with him.

Michael often writes people think of Parkinson's disease as simply having tremors. He points out it is much worse. To be frozen from diminishment of movement.

I write that people think Alzheimer's as forgetfulness, dementia, and loss of self. My prior three books try to show it's not all that bad. AZ is inexorable, and there is no cure, but there are years of mild cognitive impairment that don't prevent having a full life with pleasure and joy. As I always write: memory is not all it is cracked out to be.

On page 110, Michael writes, "If you don't take risks, there is no room for luck." I like that, but in my New Yorker contrarian way, that includes a chance for bad luck. However, in my fourth year of AZ, I am willing to take more chances. I entered into the costly ReCODE program. Now I read about a promising new drug entering into phase 3 trials.

"Lilly's donanemab works as an active immunotherapy designed to stimulate the patient's immune system to attack and destroy beta amyloid plaques that are believed to form in the brain and spur the memory-wasting disease."

We made reservations for two months in Europe next summer since the COVID-19 vaccine has come out. I'm not sure I want to forgo those plans.

On page 114 is Michael's anagnorisis.

I learned this word on Word Genius this week and wondered how I would ever use this word I never heard before. Here is the definition: "The point in a play, novel, etc., in which a principal character recognizes or discovers another character's true identity or the true nature of their own circumstances."

Michael expresses a new circumstance of his usual optimistic attitude. "I've always been confident, positive, doggedly determined; but doubt is beginning to mitigate my conviction."

On page 160: "Have I oversold hope as a panacea … My optimism is suddenly finite."

On page 186: "The third fear is like an inner minefield that you traverse as you identify, accept and process truths—such as the inexorable advance of middle age and beyond. It's the realization that we all have an expiration date, secret but certain."

On page 187: "In the same 'nothing to fear' speech, Franklin D. Roosevelt also said, 'Only a foolish optimist can deny the dark realities of the moment.'"

Michael writes, "I accept the optimism part, but now, I also admit to its foolishness."

I wonder why Michael has not started an antidepressant?

He seems to help himself with acceptance of his situation. This is the point of anagnorisis for Michael. "While you won't die from Parkinsonism, you will die with it. Complications from the disease such as the diminished ability to swallow can lead to aspirating food or pneumonia" (p. 201).

Finally, Michael comes to realize he can't golf anymore. More importantly, he realizes he can't act anymore because his speech is so impaired (p. 208).

CHAPTER 5

Irony of All Ironies
January 15, 2021

We were stuck in Florida last year due to COVID-19, struggling to decide when and how to leave for Kansas as we believed Florida would become a hotspot. Now it appears we can get the COVID-19 vaccine sooner in Florida than in Kansas.

Hence, we are thinking of driving down once we get scheduled for the vaccination, unless we can get it sooner in Kansas. Next two weeks will decide it for us. Biden's speech on getting the vaccine was very hopeful. Of course, he may not get the funding from Congress. Seems he should get the funding since he controls both houses.

News flash just came in: January 15, 2021, at 12:06 p.m. CST

> When Health and Human Services Secretary Alex Azar announced this week that the federal government would begin releasing coronavirus vaccine doses held in reserve for second shots, no such reserve existed, according to state and federal officials briefed on distribution plans. The Trump administration had already begun shipping out what was available beginning at the end

of December, taking second doses directly off the manufacturing line.

Now, health officials across the country who had anticipated their extremely limited vaccine supply as much as doubling beginning next week are confronting the reality that their allocations will remain largely flat, dashing hopes of dramatically expanding access for millions of elderly people and those with high-risk medical conditions. Health officials in some cities and states were informed in recent days about the reality of the situation, while others are still in the dark.

CHAPTER 6

Living dangerously
January 16, 2021

In expectation of getting the COVID-19 vaccine, we made plans to travel to Europe this summer. We cancelled five cruises last year, and now we are roaring to get on the road again.

We will leave NYC to Southampton on Cunard *Queen Mary 2*. Then we will go to Scotland for a Tauck tour. We fly from Glasgow to Bergen, Norway, for a Viking cruise around Great Britain and Ireland. After that, we will go to Bordeaux, France, to go on two Viking river cruises.

Some family members still think we should wait to see how effective the vaccine will be. I believe I will only have a 5 percent chance of getting sick. The influenza vaccine has worked very well for me as a physician. I still plan to wear my mask much of the time and wash my hands even more than usual while on a cruise. We should find out if the vaccine is not as good as expected by June.

CHAPTER 7

How Can I Measure if My Alzheimer's Is Getting Worse?
January 21, 2021

Today was full of accomplishments.

1- It took me a month to finally call AAA to change my car battery.
2- Today I drove for the first time since January 20, 2020.
3- I picked up a prescription at the drive-through.
4- I went to get my blood work done.

I still have some items I have procrastinated for a long time to get done.

Get my scale fixed. First attempt failed.

Get Best Buy to return the DVD I sent in to be fixed a year ago.

This past month has been full of political news. Yesterday, I watched more of the Presidential Inauguration than ever before in my life. I know more about politics now than ever before. Of course, I remember very little of what I learned in college after reading the *Federalist Papers*.

Hence, on some levels, I am smarter than I was when my diagnosis of AZ was made in December 2017.

I have actually done better on my MOCA (Montreal Cognitive Assessment). I made up my own test that I failed every day, the TOCA (Topeka Cognitive Assessment). I wrote about it in my last book. For example, what are we having for dinner?

I do think I am slowly and mildly getting worse, but it is very difficult to quantify. My wife agrees with this. I decided to choose things I do well and see when I no longer can do.

1- Taking my fifteen medicines and supplements
2- Driving
3- Cooking breakfast and lunch for myself
4- Making my evening cocktail, which involves several steps, Manhattan and Old-Fashioned
5- Getting lost on my walk

I am now hopeful I can maintain my present mental state for another three years. We just made plans to go to Europe for two months.

CHAPTER 8

Alpha-Lipoic Acid
March 12, 2021

I have done well over the last six weeks on ashwagandha. It was a big step away from traditional medicine to take this step with Dr. Bredesen's ReCODE. I do believe I am calmer with it and my sleep is deeper.

Yesterday, I met with my Atma doctor and asked what medicine I should take next. I suggested Lipoic acid, and he agreed. I purchased some on the internet today.

He liked my strategy with Omega-3 oils. He already knew that krill oil has smaller doses of DHA, but by taking 3,000 mg of Lovaza, I will still get good doses of DHA. The reason to take krill oil is to get the DHA in my blood (which is at a good level) past the blood-brain barrier.

Insights on the Use of α-Lipoic Acid for Therapeutic Purposes
Bahare Salehi
Free PMC Article

Abstract:

α-lipoic acid (ALA, thioctic acid) has various properties, among them great antioxidant potential and is widely used for diabetic polyneuropathy-associated pain and paresthesia. Naturally, ALA is located in mitochondria, where it is used as a cofactor for pyruvate dehydrogenase (PDH) and α-ketoglutarate dehydrogenase complexes. Despite its various potentials, ALA therapeutic efficacy is relatively low due to its pharmacokinetic profile. Data suggests that ALA has a short half-life and bioavailability (about 30%) triggered by its hepatic degradation, reduced solubility as well as instability in the stomach. However, the use of various innovative formulations has greatly improved ALA bioavailability.

The R enantiomer of ALA shows better pharmacokinetic parameters, including increased bioavailability as compared to its S enantiomer.

To understand how this works or looks, imagine that a clock and a pole. ... Because the 4th highest priority atom is placed in the back, the arrow should appear like it is going across the face of a clock. If it is going clockwise, then it is an R-enantiomer; If it is going counterclockwise, it is an S-enantiomer.

Indeed, the use of amphiphilic matrices has capability to improve ALA bioavailability and intestinal absorption. Also, ALA's liquid formulations are associated with greater plasma concentration and bioavailability as compared to its solidified dosage form. Thus, improved formulations can increase both ALA absorption and bioavailability, leading to a raise in therapeutic efficacy. Interestingly, ALA bioavailability will be dependent on age, while no difference has been found for gender. The present review aims to provide an update on studies from preclinical to clinical trials assessing ALA's usages in diabetic patients with neuropathy, obesity, central nervous system-related diseases and abnormalities in pregnancy. (2019 Aug. 9;9(8):356. doi: 10.3390/biom9080356)

I started ALA on March 22, 2021.

CHAPTER 9

Predicting How Many Good
Years I Will Have
March 17, 2021

I read an article in the *LA Times* about two Alzheimer's patients that recently died. Both were in nursing homes. One lady was seventy-one years old and the other was seventy-two years old. Their diagnosis was made in 2014. My diagnosis of Alzheimer's was made in December 2017. I am sixty-nine years old. I am pleased I have done so well since my diagnosis. Looking at these two ladies, I am hoping I will do well into my seventh year since diagnosis.

These ladies were in a nursing home. One lady loved gospel music. The other lady loved seeing her husband every day.

COVID-19 changed all that.

Shutdown prevented continued socialization with people from outside the nursing home. The isolation apparently caused a rapid decline in their condition. One lady died from COVID-19. The other died from Alzheimer's—probably from not eating?

I suspect their diagnosis was not made early in the course of their disease. My diagnosis was made early with mild cognitive impairment. I have become more hopeful, especially as I am trying traveling again this summer to Europe. I have Zoom calls with groups twice a week, have a new exercise bike to maintain zone 2 levels for long periods of time, do more weight lifting, continue nutritional ketosis, have very low cholesterol levels, have systolic blood pressure less than 120, keep my Hgb A1C less than 7.5, and continue my multiple medications and supplements.

1. Ramipril for diabetes, but it lowers my blood pressure.
2. Diltiazem for atrial fibrillation, but it lowers my blood pressure.

I think having a great blood pressure is important for my prognosis. Sudden decline with Alzheimer's may occur with stroke.

3. Invokana for lowering my glucose.
4. Metformin for my diabetes.
5. Xarelto for anticoagulation with my atrial fibrillation.
6. Citalopram for mild depression.
7. Ashwagandha for mood—*new* recently.
8. Magnesium threonate for helping sleep.
9. Melatonin to have regular sleep patterns.
10. CPAP machine to prevent low oxygen during sleep.
11. Vitamin D
12. Omega-3 fish oil with a fatty meal.
13. Lipitor, 10 mg day
14. Nicotinic acid, 1,000 mg (Endur-Acin)
15. Namzaric

Recently more supplements due to ReCODE protocol from *The End of Alzheimer's* book.

16. Methyl vitamin B mouth spray
17. Zinc

18. Thryve probiotics

I obtained hearing aids. I had cataract surgery.

There is no cure for Alzheimer's.

Need true grit and fortitude to keep your health as good as possible.

CHAPTER 10

Annual Visit to Florida Neurologist
March 23, 2021

I have three neurologists. Dr. Elliott made my diagnosis in December 2017.

Dr. Swerdlow is my KUMC Research Center neurologist. He entered me into my nontreatment study. I have had three years of scans with the study but I am not told the results.

Dr. Elliott gave me some good news. There should be an IV infusion given once a month to take away the amyloid plaques.

I am thinking I will continue all the ReCODE medication I am already taking. I told Dr. Elliott about my subdural. He was very concerned as I am on an anticoagulant. I told him about my festination. He did a foot-tapping test with which I did poorly.

He then stood behind me and did a pull test to see how quickly recovered. It was clear to him I was having problems similar to Parkinsonism, which I don't have, but enough neurons have been compromised by my Alzheimer's to cause similar symptoms.

He asked me to walk in the pool thirty minutes three times a week. This year he didn't do a MOCA, as he felt it wasn't sensitive enough.

I told him I have more extensive testing at KUMC Memory Center. He asked me to send me the results of those tests.

I remember when I had a finger-tapping test at one cognitive test in 2017. I thought I had done well. The tester said eighty-year-old men could do better.

The big news is a new drug coming out this June.

CHAPTER 11

Trip to Boston to Visit Grandsons
April 17, 2021

On the back cover of my year 1 book in my Alzheimer's series, I have a photo of me holding my first grandson. Last week, I visited him and his new brother, who was born this year. COVID-19 prevented us from visiting them till now. We completed our vaccinations and flew up to see them.

The baby was happy and a joy for my wife to hold. I enjoyed the two-and-a-half-year-old as he talks and interacts very well. I loved reading to him at night. I have a third grandson back in Kansas, which we have already visited. He is just a few months older than the baby in Boston. He is the happiest baby I have ever seen in my life.

I am blessed.

My short-term memory continues to get worse, but happiness and love grows.

My walking and balance has gotten worse, as I neglect to do balance exercises as well as weight lifting. I still walk five to ten thousand steps a day along the beach. Traveling to Boston interrupted my routine. Not a good excuse, since our hotel had a nice gym and pool.

I did what my neurologist prescribed after my last visit. He wanted me to go thirty minutes in the pool three times a week. I doubted I could do thirty minutes, but I was able to do fifteen minutes. It was more difficult than I thought it would be as I ploughed hard into the water.

The big surprise was that I pulled a right hip muscle. It was a setback to my exercise program due to the pain and stiffness of the hip. I continued walking at least.

Here I am in the fourth month of the year, and I have done very poorly with my weight lifting. What I continue to do exceptionally well, even while traveling, is to take my ten prescription meds in the morning, my two injections each week, and my five supplements each day. I take three pills at bedtime, which have helped my sleep—Melatonin, Magnesium threonate, and Ashwagandha.

I am pleased with the results of the Ashwagandha, which I take twice a day. I do believe it calms me.

The loss of short-term memory doesn't worry me. Memory is not it is all cracked out to be, as I have said before.

What bothers me is how quickly I can get angry, especially with my wife. If we continue to argue, I get very distressed and depressed.

My wife is a wonderful caretaker and person, but there are certain deficits in my personality that she wishes me to improve on. To me, of course, they are trivial. I endeavor to do better.

Her pet peeves are as follows:

1. Spilling food and drink on my shirt.

2. Her new car getting seeds on the seat when we drove down to Florida last month. The seeds are very difficult to vacuum up.
3. In general, I am a slob and always have been.
4. She prefers to drive and will get angry at me for trying to help her with back-seat driver suggestions.

On the drive down from Kansas, I did drive a couple of hours a day to give her some relief. I try to keep quiet when she is driving, but she does appreciate my help on the GPS driving directions.

5. Overall she has trained me well.

She has no idea how any unkindness from anyone affects my mood so badly. I have been very sensitive.

I already take an antidepressant, but it doesn't prevent short-term depression from stress.

CHAPTER 12

Choline
May 3, 2021

I just discovered the importance of choline from the ReCODE protocol.

I always preached that the egg was the perfect food, as it had many nonessential amino acids that our body cannot manufacture. Alzheimer's patients have lower levels of the enzyme that changes choline to acetylcholine in the brain.

This is why I have taken Namzaric for the last three years and six months. Usually, it's beneficial effect fades in trails after two years. Perhaps I have done well because I began therapy early in a mild cognitive dysfunction stage?

On Atkins, I was eating three fried eggs a day. That's 440 mg of choline a day. Males should take in 550 mg, and females should take in 450 mg.

I had cut down to two eggs a day for less calories. Now I have returned to three eggs a day for the choline. Liver is a good source as well, but I don't like the taste.

Is it maybe more important to eat more eggs early in life to prevent Alzheimer's? There is no strong evidence, and many people may worry about their cholesterol. My LDLc is thirty-eight on low dose of atorvastatin and Endur-Acin. This may be one of the main reasons I am doing better than expected with the course of my Alzheimer's. Prevention of vascular disease is very important in preventing heart attack and stroke—major reasons for sudden decline in Alzheimer's patients.

Chicken and beef also provide choline. Even though most Americans probably take less choline than suggested, clinical deficiency is rarely seen. However, by age eighty perhaps it does contribute to 50 percent of the population getting Alzheimer's.

Eat the eggs. Cooking the eggs does not decrease the level of choline in the egg.

Even if we have good levels of choline, it doesn't help AZ patients, as they have low levels of the enzyme that converts choline into acetylcholine in the brain. Take Namzaric or similar drugs.

CHAPTER 13

Update on Fish Oil Levels
May 14, 2021

I had OmegaQuant do my omega-3 levels on February 9, 2021. I had them done with the ReCODE cognoscopy earlier, but I wanted to compare their results to OmegaQuant.

I repeated OmegaQuant on May 2, 2021, as I had learned from Dr. Dale Bredensen that the brain does not make DHA omega-3. I asked my mentor lipidologist, Dr. Michael Davidson from the National Lipid Association, about it. He advised krill oil, as it has a chemical in it that carries the DHA from the blood across the blood-brain barrier to the brain, lyso-PC DHA with MSFD2a. Krill oil has the most lyso-PC DHA.

Thus, even though my two DHA levels were good in the blood, it did not mean it was crossing into the brain. Hence, I began taking two krill oil pills with a total 64 mg of EPA and 30 mg DHA, which is the advised dose on the bottle.

I decreased my omega-3 fish from four to three capsules a day. Three a day is their advised dose. I was taking 1,600 mg EPA and 1,100 mg DHA on four capsules. On three capsules, I am only taking 1,200 mg EPA and only 900 mg DHA. By replacing the one triple-strength omega-3 fish with two krill oil capsules, I had decreased my DHA and EPA intake.

I felt it was time to check my OmegaQuant levels again to see if it made a difference. I learned I can increase the absorption of omega-3s if I take them after eating a fatty meal.

On May 2, I sent in my second sample and received the results back on May 14:

> The Omega-3 Index is the proportion of long-chain omega-3s, eicosapentaenoic acid (EPA) and docosahexaenoic acid (DHA), of all fatty acids in your red blood cell membranes. It reflects the omega-3 status of your body over the last 4 months.

My omega-3 index went down a little below the desired level of 8 percent. Before, on the higher dose of omega-3 with the triple-strength pills, it was in the good range of 9.3 percent. I guess I need to go back to taking four capsules.

My DHA went from 3.63 percent to 3.37 percent. Not a significant change on a smaller dose, but with the krill oil, more DHA gets into the brain.

I know this is complicated, but this is why the subtitle of the food is *True Grit and Fortitude Required*.

CHAPTER 14

Courage
May 15, 2021

I am reading Stephen Grimble's book titled *For Love & Liberty*. It is an excellent book. The novel presents the conservative side of politics in a consistent and rational way with a depth of knowledge rarely seen on the GOP side.

So far, my favorite part was a speech about courage that jumped out at me, starting on page 270.

Excerpts and some paraphrasing.

Speech given by presidential candidate Reb at his former military school. The motto of this school is "Courage, honor, conquer." It is not by accident that courage was placed first.

Winston Churchill once said, "Courage is rightly esteemed the first of human qualities because it is the quality that guarantees all the others."

We have all heard "that person has the courage of his convictions."

Absent courage, we would have no convictions.

The courage we all have to find within ourselves day after day typically is not physical courage, but the moral courage to remain true to all other virtues and to persevere in the face of adversity. In this sense, courage is the conscious act of free will.

CHAPTER 15

Return to Kansas
May 18, 2021

Ginger just drove 1,400 miles over three days. She prefers I don't drive. During the entire drive, we listened to a Stephen King novel. I realized I could follow the narrative, but I also realized I couldn't concentrate on the story and drive at the same time.

It's a good time. CDC announced vaccinated people don't need to wear masks outdoors. We are hoping to be able to go on two Viking river cruises in France in August.

It was great to be on the beach in Florida. I walked every day and used the gym for some light weight lifting.

CHAPTER 16

Cleaning the Brain of Its Toxins?
June 13, 2021

Glymphatic circulation of the brain is thought to clean toxins out of the brain during sleep. Perhaps CST (craniosacral therapy) can also do this by increasing the flow of CSF in the brain. Craniosacral therapy is a technique all can learn in just one or two days. The flow of cerebrospinal fluid is increased. For those with Alzheimer's disease, the statistics for decreased flow of CSF are even more severe, the impairment reaches to 75 percent of a normal adult. The glymphatic system is a system for waste clearance in the central nervous system of vertebrates.

CHAPTER 17

A Tattoo on My Brain Review: Part I
June 23, 2021

I began reading a book by a neurologist with Alzheimer's written in the first person (mostly?), also written with Teresa H. Barker (ghostwriter?). I am really into this book.

This neurologist was diagnosed with Alzheimer's two years before I was. On page 72, Dr. Gibbs writes about his mental status at age sixty-three.

His cognitive status seems worse than my present mental status at age sixty-nine and seven months. Like me, Dr. Gibbs believes it is important to be diagnosed with Alzheimer's as early as possible. When I received *A Tattoo on My Brain* yesterday, I started as I usually do by going to the index at the back.

In the index, I looked for the following:

1. Ketosis.
2. Statins.
3. Alcohol (see #5).
4. Cholesterol level and heart attacks.

5. Supplements (only one I found was flavonols, p. 129). He does not seem to advise dark chocolate but does advise citrus, apples, legumes, berries, and red wine.
6. Medicinal herbs were found on page 123. Dr. Gibbs entered a trial to measure levels of this herb with a washout period. He never stated the name of the herb.
7. Dr. Richard Isaacson and Dr. Dale Bredensen were not in the index.
8. Lab work results.
9. Death from time of diagnosis, page 12? Eight years with no change since the first patient was diagnosed.
10. Dreams, page 162.

What I really love about this book is Dr. Gibbs writes in the first person about his journey with Alzheimer's. I found someone I can compare my own progress with Alzheimer's.

There are others, such as Bredesen's Julia and Isaacson's poster child, but they have not written a detailed memoir such as Dr. Gibbs and myself.

Dr. Gibbs is homozygous positive for ApoE4 gene. I have only one gene for it. Dr. Gibbs never describes himself as having early onset AZ. One of my neurologists said I had early onset, which surprised me. Perhaps because we know the disease does have an asymptomatic phase ten to twenty years earlier, which I did suspect for myself.

Dr. Gibbs's mental reserve is clearly gigantic compared to mine. His level of education and scientific research over the years is impressive. I seem to be doing better than he did. I suggest it is because of the following:

1. I am in ketosis with Atkins diet.
2. I keep my systolic blood pressure less than 100 with two drugs: ramipril (for DM) and diltiazem (for a fib).

3. I keep my LDLp down to 300 (rock bottom).
4. I keep my nonfasting triglycerides less than 100.
5. I am still able to write my books yearly, which I think keeps me mentally sharp.

CHAPTER 18

A Tattoo on My Brain Review: Part II
June 23, 2021

It was 229 pages long, and I received it on June 8. The last three days, I pushed myself to finish it so that I could start reviewing it in detail.

Introduction

"It's [AZ] slowly growing presence in my brain."

"In the most universal sense a diagnosis of AZ is clarifying, it presents the uninvited opportunity."

"A definitive diagnosis of Alzheimer's requires evidence of Amyloid plaques."

"When we realized in early 2019 that the conversation about Alzheimer's had long been stuck on fast-forward to the late stage."

CHAPTER 19

A Tattoo on My Brain Review: Part III
June 24, 2021

Prologue

On page 12: "More than 100 years since Auguste's diagnosis [first patient diagnosed with Alzheimer's] and death. And yet the typical time from diagnosis to death for those with Alzheimer's has remained the same, about EIGHT YEARS."

CHAPTER 20

The Smell of Baking Bread

Thirteen years ago was Dr. Gibbs's first sign of AZ (p. 27).

"False odors are called phantosmias."

Dr. Gibbs's internist had him get an MRI, which he didn't think he needed. It turned out the MRI showed a pineal gland tumor. The tumor was large enough to press on his optic nerve, but so far, it did not affect his vision. The benign tumor was removed uneventfully.

A stubborn puzzle (p. 39).

The neurosurgeon "had never seen a pituitary tumor … cause loss of smell" (p. 61).

By the beginning of 2013, "by most standards I was still cognitively normal."

At age sixty-two, he was concerned by nagging with recall of names and words, and he was homozygous for ApoE4 for AZ (p. 64).

About a year after retiring as 1964 began, he went to a dementia specialist for formal cognitive assessment. Results were normal except for delayed verbal recall which gave him the diagnosis of mild cognitive impairment (MCI) (p. 75).

In 2015, his cognitive test was unchanged except for a high score on depression. Dr. Gibbs doesn't discuss if he went on antidepressants (p. 83).

September 2015, "there were the unmistakable tell-tale signs of Alzheimer's on the Amyloid Pet Scan and the Tau Pet scan" (p. 87).

Dr. Gibbs's cognitive scores were better than could be expected based on his scans. Dr. Gibbs suggested that "lifetime habits of study and stretching to learn and other stimulating cognitive activity, contribute to so-called cognitive reserve, a kind of brain bank of neural cells or networks that provided back up, or created resilience, that might be keeping my cognitive function high despite the presence of brain atrophy and accumulations of plaques and tangles normally seen in mild to moderate Alzheimer's disease."

CHAPTER 21

A Tattoo on My Brain Review: Part IV
June 25, 2021

"A recent study reported in JAMA Neurology showed that high cognitive reserve, as measured by education and high baseline intelligence, DOES NOT protect from Tau-associated brain atrophy but it DOES lead to a delay in cognitive impairment, postponing the onset of of the symptoms of Alzheimer's disease" (p. 91).

"There's no way yet to measure cognitive reserve" (p. 96).

"In March 2016, I [Dr. Gibbs] entered a phase 3 clinical trial of the antibody called aducanumab" (p. 102). Three positive points about this new drug: "First ... was based on a naturally occurring antibody found in the blood of elderly people who did not have any cognitive impairment ... Second, side effects appeared minimal."

ARIA (amyloid related imaging abnormalities). "Most of the patients with ARIA had no symptoms at all," and third, "the results of the earlier phase one trial looked very encouraging" (p. 109)

Chapter 13 is the most important and climatic chapter in the book. At the end of September 2017, Dr. Gibbs had his first infusion of aducanumab. No side effects.

Next month after the second infusion, he experiences a new phantosmia. A week after the third infusion, the headaches began.

"On December 13, about six weeks into this treatment period I started having trouble reading simple words ... About a week later, late one evening, my headache suddenly exploded with excruciating pain." Admitted to ICU, he had an MRI which showed "many areas of brain swelling and micro-hemorrhages ... these were classic imaging findings of ARIA."

"Repeat MRI a month later showed the brain swelling was actually a little worse despite not getting any more infusions of the test drug." Dr. Gibbs was the first trial participate who required treatment for the side effects of aducanumab. His side effects were considered "unique and concerning."

Dr. Gibbs's "doctors decided to treat it as they would a serious flare-up of multiple sclerosis (MS)." Treatment was "five daily infusions of very high dose steroids."

"After the third day my headaches went away and I was able to read again ... By the summer of 2018, I was feeling really good."

CHAPTER 22

A Tattoo on My Brain Review: Part V
June 25, 2021

"Most of the conversation about Alzheimer's is about fear and loss and things you can't or eventually won't be able to do, or do anything about. Helplessness and hopelessness have been the dominant theme of the conversation for more than a century" (p. 125).

"In short, the science suggests when the sense of smell goes missing, it can disrupt the mechanism for making and retrieving memories" (p. 144).

"Multiple types of complex brain processing of sensory information can be inpaired by Alzheimer's, some in the early stages and some later in the disease. A remarkable exception is music" (p. 147).

CHAPTER 23

A Tattoo on My Brain Review: Part VI
June 26, 2021

Chapter 16 in *A Tattoo on My Brain*: "It's only scary if you look down."

I came to understand this chapter better after reading it a second time.

Dr. Gibbs speaks about a patient with forgetfulness that he told she may have early Alzheimer's, but there was no way to know for certain. A month later, he found out she committed suicide.
When I first learned I had Alzheimer's, confirmed by a PET Amyloid scan in December 2017, I was bewildered because I had no idea of my prognosis. The best I could hope for was two years of a steady course on Namzaric. I thought about my diagnosis most of the day. This is why I titled my first book *I Am Waiting For When I Forget I Have Alzheimer's*.

Dr. Gibbs writes on page 158, "Someone's fear of the future as they come to terms with the diagnosis can often be debilitating beyond the burden of the physical disease itself."

This is why I write and publish a yearly journal of the course of my Alzheimer's. I am seven months into the writing of my fourth year since my diagnosis was made. I hope the details of my journey will make it clear to someone that if you make the diagnosis early when you only have mild cognitive impairment, you probably have a good many years ahead of you.

As Dr. Gibbs writes on page 168, "One thing that is striking as you get near the top of Beacon Rock is to look down at the boat dock below. The boats tied to it are so tiny you can barely make them out. Looking down isn't always scary. It can also heighten your sense of gain in altitude. You can feel how far you have come."

After forty-three months of living a wonderful life with Alzheimer's, I can certainly understand and agree with Dr. Gibbs's above statement.

CHAPTER 24

Diets for Early Alzheimer's
June 25, 2021

There are various books' opinions on diet for Alzheimer's.

Mind Diet

1. *A Tattoo on My Brain* by Dr. Gibbs
2. *Keep Sharp: Build a Better Brian at Any Age* by Dr. Gupta
3. Mayo Clinic's MIND diet, short for Mediterranean-DASH intervention for Neurodegenerative
4. Ketosis diet

The End of Alzheimer's by Dr. Dale Bredensen

KetoFLEX 12/3, p. 179

"You can follow principles as a vegetarian or omnivore and get the same benefits."

"Mild ketosis … is optimal for cognitive function."

"Combine a low carbohydrate diet with 12-hour overnight fast."

(*The Alzheimer's Antidote* by Amy Berger, p. 27)

"Two points are clear. AZ is at least in part exacerbated by chronic progressive brain fuel starvation due to specifically to brain glucose deficit and attempting to treat the cognitive deficit early in AZ using ketogenic interventions in clinical trials is safe, clinical, ethical, and scientifically well founded" (Stephen Cunnane)

CHAPTER 25

Amazon Review of *A Tattoo on My Brain*
June 30, 2021

This is the best book I have read on Alzheimer's. First, it is written in the first person (with ghostwriter). Second, it is very timely. Dr. Gibbs was first to have a reaction from aducanumab that put him in ICU. He recovered from ARIA with high dose IV steroids. Amazing that he improved his mentation to the point where he thinks he is better than before the aducanumab.

As a physician, I found his expertise as a neurologist very informative. Others might find it too much in the weeds.

I am only giving him 4.5 stars because he does not discuss keto diet or going on statins to get cholesterol down as low as possible to avoid stroke and heart attack. These are two events that can cause an Alzheimer's to "fall off a cliff."

The rest of his advice is fairly standard. But it is his personal writing that gave me so much solace and so much for me to hope for myself as I am in my fourth year of having Alzheimer's.

CHAPTER 26

Update on a New AZ Drug
July 9, 2021

I am eligible for Aduhelm IV infusions. I know I have a great deal of amyloid in my brain. I am doing well with Dr. Dale Bredesen's ReCODE protocol, which tries to decrease inflammation that they believe causes the formation of amyloid. The ReCODE protocol is expensive but not as bad as the cost of the IV infusion at this point. Thus, I will wait another six months for the post trial results to come in and see how insurance coverage goes.

Thus, I may wait too long.

I think the sudden drop in function is usually due to vascular reasons. Since my cholesterol is extremely low and my systolic blood pressure is usually under 120, I think my chances of falling off a cliff are low.

It's time for the media to take a close look at the choices for someone with mild cognitive impairment

Early Alzheimer's

1. New approved drug aducanumab
2. Multifaceted approach with Dr. Dale Bredesen's ReCODE protocol
3. Multifaceted approach with Dr. Richard Isaacson's protocol.

Review of Peter Attia's Podcast

Three points of good news on all these fronts.

1. Aducanumab

In Dr. Gibbs's personal experience, getting ARIA with the new drug and treating the inflammation with high dose steroids may be the best new approach.

2. Dr. Bredesen's ReCODE Protocol

I was very skeptical of the long list of nostrums for AZ. However, COVID-19 occurred, and I had the time and the money to pursue this program. I was most interested in getting their cognoscopy lab work ($500). I paid for a one-year appointment for around $2,500. Higher prices in bigger cities.

3. Dr. Isaacson's Protocol

It has been difficult to find out what is in his Cornell protocol. I suspect it is similar to Dr. Bredesen's protocol. No idea what the cost is to go to his clinic in NYC. I have his and Dr. Chris Ochner's book: *The Alzheimer's Prevention and Treatment Diet: Using Nutrition to Combat the Effects of Alzheimer's Disease.*

It is comforting to see two independent Alzheimer's experts with good results in their programs.

All these choices are expensive. They all have a similar basic approach that can be started immediately without expensive supplements.

1. Exercise
2. Sleep
3. Different healthy diets, proposed list of three diets
4. Socialization
5. Control blood pressure
6. Lower cholesterol
7. Treat diabetes
8. Try to maintain a healthy weight

What will motivate you to do that lengthy list? Make the diagnosis early! Go to a neurologist that has an interest in dementia.

After he does the usual tests and labs to exclude a possible secondary (treatable) cause of dementia, ask him/her to refer you to a cognitive psychologist who specializes with three-hour testing. So far, this is the only way to pick up Alzheimer's early.

With an amyloid PET scan, I was finally diagnosed in December 2017. I was immediately started on Namzaric.

CHAPTER 27

Memory Is Not What It's Cracked Out to Be

July 2021

If it's mostly short-term memory.

I show hope for people with early Alzheimer's.

I was able to add fifty-five capitals of the fifty-five European nations to my memory palace I made a couple of years ago. I use my memory palace if I have trouble falling asleep. Sometimes I fall asleep before I finish the first five smallest European nations. It must be like a hypnotic suggestion. Since I travel so much and meet many fellow travelers on cruises, I find it useful to have this information about Europe.

CHAPTER 28

National Weight Control Registry Survey
July 11, 2021

Today, I took the survey with the news that I finally broke through my plateau. I didn't change my exercise or my ketosis with the Atkins diet. What I did was increase Ozempic from 0.5 mg to 1.0 mg. It decreased my appetite, which allowed me to decrease my calorie intake. I was running at 210 pounds but have finally dropped to 199 pounds. I often cannot eat a whole meal, especially the meat.

I have proposed my sponge theory to Dr. Rosenbaum. Weight regain occurs due to the fact that fat cells don't disappear with weight loss. They shrink, and the low leptin levels cause weight to regain due to hunger and low metabolic rates. He didn't seem to give it much credit.

Now my plateau has reset due to Ozempic.

If my brain tries to reset, I will have the option of going on higher dose with Wegovy 2.6 mg.

I suspect if I can't increase my dose or eventually have less response to the high dose, I will go back to a higher plateau as predicted by Dr. Rosenbaum.

CHAPTER 29

Life Goes On Even with Alzheimer's
Monday, July 12, 2021

"Ob-La-Di, Ob-La-Da" has been ridiculed by some commentators for its lightheartedness. From 2009, McCartney has regularly performed the song in concert.

Today, this song has more significance for me.

In December 2017, I was diagnosed with AZ and started on Namzaric. There was no cure. Even with the new drug Aduhelm, today there is no cure. I was hopeful I would have two more years with Namzaric. Now, I don't think my mentation is worse after

Three years and eight months have passed. This is why I have written three books on my Alzheimer's, showing my progress.

- *I Am Waiting For When I Forget I Have Alzheimer's: Year One*
- *Traveling with Alzheimer's: Year Two*
- *Pursuit of Happiness with Alzheimer's: Year Three*

I am in the middle of my fourth book titled "Alzheimer's Is Inexorable." Perhaps this doesn't sound so hopeful. My message tries to be realistic in presenting the facts in my AZ journey, and with the onset of the COVID-19 pandemic this past year I have fallen into a routine, which I believed helped me.

"Ob-la-di, ob-la-da, life goes on, bra, / oh how the life goes on."

How very true.

I had a concussion and subdural hematoma from head trauma. My walking became worse with falls due to festination. My depression became worse after the concussion. I increased my Citalopram. I treated my anxiety with pacing. However, my anger was a major problem for me and my marriage.

Anger.

We worked out a process with a safe word: *promise.*

On my visit to my KUMC memory neurologist last month, I complained to him about my wife always getting after me about picking up and not spilling food on myself. The neurologist simply said that is what wives do. I said, "Doc, she is not in the room right now, you don't have to say this." It did not change his opinion.

We have done better. I think maybe she is not so overloaded. She had the house renovated and has chronic pain due to too much housework. We had made a promise to each other that if the conversation turned angry, we could shut it down with the safe word.

These were all major advancements for me. It all begs the question, did Dr. Dale Bredesen's ReCODE protocol make a difference?

I will subtitle my next book "True Grit and Fortitude Required."

I usually go to bed around 10:00 to 11:00 p.m. Usually wake up around 9:30 a.m. I get up to urinate three times a night but have no trouble going back to sleep. My Fitbit says I average eight hours sleep a night. I made a major change when I started three medications at night.

1. Magnesium L-threonate, 4,000 mg
2. Ashwagandha
3. Melatonin, 5 mg

The only side effect I have is a mild transient esophageal reflux. My real Ob-la-di routine starts when I wake up. I weigh myself on my BIA scale. I recently broke my plateau and weighed 199.5 lbs. with the help of increasing my weekly injection of Ozempic from 0.5 mg to 1.0. I check my fasting glucose and ketone level daily and record it. I also take 100 mg testosterone injections each week. This, along with weekly Cialis, allows me to continue a sex life.

Morning prescription medications:

1. Thryve probiotic, 2 tabs
2. Citalopram, 2 tabs
3. Metformin, 4 tabs (500 mg each)
4. DHEA, 10 mg (2 tabs)
5. Atorvastatin, 10 mg
6. Endur-Acin, 500 mg (2 tabs) (nicotinic acid)
7. Xarelto (1 tab)
8. Namzaric (1 tab)
9. Ramipril, 10 mg
10. Cardizem, 360 mg
11. I take a morning pill of Ashwagandha (I do think this may have helped me to be calmer).

I make my morning coffee with 93 percent Lindt dark chocolate to get flavonoids. I usually drink two cups of coffee to get antioxidants. I will drink a diet Coke each morning to help move my bowels. I take two sprays of Liposomal Methyl B Complex under my tongue. I put off breakfast till 11:00 a.m. or till 1:00 p.m. I take turmeric twice a day after my meals.

My first meal of the day is a choice of three high-fat meals:

1. Two eggs and two slices bacon (if lucky, wife adds spinach).
2. High-grain English muffin (100 calories) with cream cheese on one side and butter on the other side. I jazz it up with capers on the cream cheese and Everything Bagel salt.

I recently added some salmon slices to the cream cheese.

3. Some English muffin, but with peanut butter that I roast in a toaster oven. I then put two slices of bacon on it.

I take my omega-3 after a fatty meal to increase absorption.

- Krill oil, 500 mg; EPA, 64 mg; DHA, 30mg (two tabs)
- Omega-3 triple strength, 1,200 EPA + 900 DHA (3 capsules)

I usually anchor my day with a Manhattan cocktail around 3:00 p.m. I have a small bag of pistachios with it.

I try to put dinner off till after 7:00 p.m. I take evening supplements:

- Zinc picolinate, 22 mg a day
- Alpha-lipoic acid, 2 tabs (600 mg)
- Vitamin D3, 4,000 units

I usually walk a mile each day (twenty minutes) up and down a good-sized hill in the afternoon.

After dinner, I ride my Keiser stationary bike for twenty minutes at an easy pace after I have done my stretching on the floor. I also do ten to fifteen dumbbell curls with ten pounds in each hand. I go up and down the stairs ten times a day.

I am amazed I have a system to remember to take all these pills each day. I rarely screw up. As long as I can continue this executive function, I don't worry that my short-term memory gets worse.

CHAPTER 30

Minor Staircase Disaster
Sunday, July 25, 2021

I missed the last step on my basement staircase and dropped a tray with plates and glasses. Another result of my Alzheimer's—poor balance.

I haven't fallen on my daily one-mile walk since I purchased a cane. I have fallen on the steps before. This time because I was carrying a heavy tray, I went one step at a time. At the end, I hit my elbow as I tried to navigate a bend in the staircase, and down it all went despite my best efforts on mindfulness. I usually divide the load and make more trips. That way I can hold two glasses in my right hand while using one or two fingers to hold on the right banister. This time, after a party, my wife had loaded the tray, and I just went for it—a mistake I will try not to make again. Haste makes waste.

CHAPTER 31

Executive Function Challenge
July 26, 2021

I passed an executive function challenge today. I was babysitting the three Newfie dogs while my wife was at a rehab appointment. While flossing my teeth, I pulled out a temporary cap on my tooth. I called the dentist, and the receptionist said my permanent cap came in early, and if I came in right now, she could fit me in. I said, "Let me call you back after I clear it with my wife."

My wife had thirty minutes left in her therapy. She told me the dogs should be okay on their own, and she would get back as soon as she could. I jumped in the car and drove to the dentist. I paced the hall for fifteen minutes waiting for my turn. Right now, I have 4,500 steps on Fitbit. It was a simple procedure. It was very smooth and efficient. They gave me the mold for the gold tooth.

This may all seem mundane, but I was dx'd with AZ in December 2017. My short-term memory continues to get worse, but I was able to make the executive functions described above.

CHAPTER 32

I Enjoy My Mornings
July 28, 2021

I try to count my blessings after three years and eight months since my diagnosis of Alzheimer's. My first year was filled with anxiety, as I had no idea what my prognosis was. That is why I titled my first-year book *I Am Waiting For When I Forget I Have Alzheimer's*. I was counseled to just have fun. Thus, in my second-year book, *Traveling with Alzheimer's*, I continued in my third-year book, *The Pursuit of Happiness with Alzheimer's*. In the third year, due to COVID-19, we had to cancel five cruises.

Again trying to find a silver lining, I concentrated on new ways to approach my disease:

1. Intermittent fasting.
2. Started Dr. Dale Bredesen's ReCODE program at Atma Holistic Clinic.
3. I slowly began adding supplements that they advised. I take about ten new ones.
4. I am writing my fourth year book now to be titled "Alzheimer's Is Inexorable: True Grit and Fortitude Required."

It requires a great deal of discipline to follow the rigorous routine of diet, exercise, and medications. It is expensive. So why do I continue to do it? I clearly feel better. Maybe not cognitively, but emotionally. My anxiety is much less. I don't pace as much as I did. I still have some mounting anxiety as the day progresses—worse if I get into an argument with my wife. The most beautiful part is the tranquility of my mornings. I try not to schedule any appointments before noon. I go to bed around 9:00 to 10:00 p.m. and have rediscovered Bernard Cornwell's historic novels. I take melatonin, Mg L-threonate, and Ashwagandha. After about forty minutes of reading, I easily go to sleep.

It is a good, deep sleep with many dreams. I usually go through a sleep cycle of 75 to 120 minutes before my bladder asks me to take care of it. I have no trouble going back to sleep. I wake up around 8:00 to 9:00 a.m., but I find I can still sleep another hour or two, and I do. I take time to get myself out of bed because my body and mind feel excellent. Serenity, no pain. I lie there and just enjoy the moment. Then I get up and start my routine with joy and anticipation. I think Atma's supplements have something to do with it.

One problem may be that spending twelve hours in bed can cause sarcopenia. I average more than eight hours of sleep each night on my Fitbit and Apple watch. I walk at least five thousand steps a day. I try to ride my stationary bike twenty minutes a day. I do curls with low weights (fifteen repetitions).

CHAPTER 33

Takeaways from Bredesen's Podcast on Fasting
July 30, 2021

Cinnamon to Lower Glucose

I may have reversed my insulin resistance when I lost 80 lbs. over a year with a low-calorie diet and exercise. However, I gained back 50 lbs. over the following year after my marriage in June 2007 despite two and a half hours of exercise a day. I ate more fruit because I thought it was a healthy form of glucose. Problem is I ate too many cherries.

Started Atkins Diet

Despite losing the 50 lbs. I had gained back and exercising, I was still insulin resistant. Listening to Dr. Bredesen's podcast on fasting with his coauthor and AZ survivor, I was surprised that they thought I could still reverse my insulin resistance.

That might be true if I got down to my prior low weight of 200 lbs. after the wedding. I hoped to lose enough central belly fat that I could improve my adiponectin level. That has not happened. There is a final role of fat that I just can't seem to lose.

Role of Central Fat that Seems Permanent

I suspect if I get cancer, I might lose that role of fat, but I will also suffer from severe sarcopenia (loss of muscle). I have been in nutritional ketosis since I started Atkins around 2015. My levels are almost always over 0.5, and lately, they are usually over 2.0 AM.

In the *End of Alzheimer's Program*, on page 32, it states, "Restoring insulin sensitivity can be achieved by" the following:

1. KetoFLEX 12/3 diet
2. Key nutrient—zinc
3. Exercise
4. Reduce stress
5. Treat sleep apnea (I'm on CPAP)

And if needed:

6. Berberine
7. Cinnamon
8. Alpha-lipoic acid (started a couple of months ago)
9. Chromium picolinate

"Virtually all of us can become insulin sensitive using this approach."

I find this to be a very bold claim. I have done most of the above.

Now I am willing to add cinnamon.

CHAPTER 34

Climbing the Bredesen ReCODE Supplement Ladder
August 1, 2021

Alpha-GPC for Cognition + Benefits, Dosage & Side Effects
Written by Aleksa Ristic, MS (Pharmacy) | Reviewed by Ana
Aleksic, MSc (Pharmacy) | Last updated: July 30, 2020

Alpha-GPC is a crucial component for the brain and a popular nootropic supplement.

It may boost mental and physical performance and supply choline to protect the nerves. Still, clinical research supports only a fraction of promoted supplementation benefits.

Choline from alpha-GPC also builds acetylcholine, a neurotransmitter that maintains your cognitive and muscle functions.

In some European countries, alpha-GPC is a prescription drug for Alzheimer's disease (Gliatilin, Delecit).

In the US, it's sold as a dietary supplement for memory enhancement.

Supplement and drug manufacturers usually derive alpha-GPC from egg or soy lecithin.

Skeptics:

* May cause headaches and digestive issues

* May increase irritability

* Not safe for children and pregnant women"

CDP-Choline vs. Alpha-GPC

Let's start with the basics. CDP-choline or citicoline is made of choline (with two phosphate groups) and cytidine, while alpha-GPC is made of choline (with one phosphate group) and glycerol.

This may sound pretty similar, but it gives rise to some interesting, distinct effects in the body [8].

For one, alpha-GPC raises choline blood levels to a greater extent than CDP-choline.

As a result, it has a more powerful impact on age-related cognitive decline and physical performance.

Secondly, alpha-GPC may stimulate fat burning and growth hormone production, giving it an edge over CDP-choline among bodybuilders [9, 10, 11,12, 13].

On the other hand, CDP-choline is essential for the production of phosphatidylcholine.

It has a broader range of active metabolites and potential benefits on mental health.

In Alzheimer's disease, bundles of mutated proteins kill neurons and deplete acetylcholine, causing an array of cognitive issues [28].

In a clinical trial of 260 patients, alpha-GPC improved all symptoms of Alzheimer's disease. In another trial of 113 patients, it boosted the effects of standard treatment (donepezil) [29, 30].

In Alzheimer's disease, bundles of mutated proteins kill neurons and deplete acetylcholine, causing an array of cognitive issues [28].

In a clinical trial of 260 patients, alpha-GPC improved all symptoms of Alzheimer's disease. In another trial of 113 patients, it boosted the effects of standard treatment (donepezil) [29, 30].

CHAPTER 35

A New Fun Experience with My Wife
August 2, 2021

My daughter and her husband purchased a SaloonBox kit for me for Father's Day. I like mixology, but the directions seemed complicated to me, so I asked my wife to help me.

I have a home bar, which I call the See No Evil bar. I make a great Manhattan each day. That is three ounces of bourbon a day.

I am doing the ReCODE protocol of Dr. Dale Bredesen for Alzheimer's. He allows some wine. Four ounces of wine is only one ounce of alcohol.

I have a nutritional therapist with Atma Clinic. I confessed to her that I have a cocktail each day, either a Manhattan or a Vodka martini. She gave me absolution. She said it anchors my day. It really does. It's a mental activity that I enjoy. I put off breakfast till 11:00 a.m., and then I put off lunch with a 2:00 p.m. happy hour. I have a small bag of pistachios with the drink. I often start a movie as well.

This SaloonBox strawberry mix took it a notch higher: more ingredients. I don't care for sweet drinks anymore, but this was good. I had my wife check me on each step of the directions, which was fun.

Father's Day was a while ago, so it took me a while to do this new challenge. My wife's willing participation was what got me out of my apathy to try something new.

I have read you should not drink five ounces or more of alcohol a day. With two glasses of red wine, I usually exceed that amount. Except for my subdural hematoma, I have not had any medical problems with drinking.

I am more careful now by drinking water between alcohol and waiting a while. I love to buy the beverage package on cruises. I never went to bars when I was young, but now I am a barfly on the cruise, as it is great socialization meeting new people. I often have ten alcoholic beverages during the day.

You can drink *all* day, if you don't start early in the morning.

I always start the day on the ocean at the baristic with an alcoholic coffee. Then wine at lunch and dinner. I have a cocktail at the bar before dinner and sometimes stop at the bar before bed.

Most people reading this must go "tsk, tsk."

1. Too much alcohol?
2. My lipid panel levels on statin are too low? LDLc 31.
3. I have been on Atkins since 2011 and in nutritional ketosis.
4. My systolic BP is usually between 90 and 120.

My reply is I have done better than expected with my AZ diagnosed in December 2017. I am down to my lowest weight since my marriage fourteen years ago, 200 pounds. I take Ozempic 1.0 mg a week, which has helped with the last ten-pound weight loss. Depression, anxiety and apathy are a big problem with Alzheimer's.

Citalopram and Ashwagandha have helped that.

People with chronic diseases such as obesity, diabetes, and AZ need to find a way to deal with it as they are the ones who with true grit and fortitude and must follow a regimen of multiple medications, supplements, diet, and exercise to try and prevent the sudden falling off of a cliff that can occur with AZ due to stroke and heart attack.

I avoid hopelessness and apathy with my cocktail anchor each day.

I am writing my fourth year book of how I have tried to enjoy my life despite the cloud of the inevitable fatal Alzheimer's hanging over my head. Each year that I finish a book, I feel a great deal of accomplishment.

I am trying to give people first-person documentation of how I am doing it with the goal that they will make their diagnosis early and realize that with mild cognitive impairment, you have several years of life ahead of you.

CHAPTER 36

The Cheapest and Easiest Way to Try to Prevent Progression of Alzheimer's
August 3, 2021

Most people can't afford $7,000 to enter a Dr. Dale Bredesen's ReCODE program. Also the supplements can cost $1,300 a year. Most people don't want to take so many pills. So what does Medicare pay for?

1. Namzaric
2. Invokana for diabetes
3. Ozempic shots for DM and weight loss
4. Metformin for DM
5. Blood pressure pills
6. Statins, Zetia
7. Testosterone
8. Citalopram

Ask your doctor which are good for you. In my opinion, these are the pills that will prevent you from suddenly falling off the cliff with Alzheimer's by a stroke or heart attack.

What supplements are needed? Vitamin D (Medicare should pay for lab test).

Which diet? Atkins or low carb, high fat diet to get into daily nutritional ketosis.

How much exercise? Exercise—this is a very individualized item. The elderly need to be careful to avoid injury. Walking twenty minutes a day is the easiest path. Then if anxious, do pacing in the house to get up to ten thousand steps. If you can do more with weights, good. I myself have cut back on weights due to some joint pain, but I try to do curls with light weights.

Some advise HIIT (high intensity interval training). I think this is fine for a younger group, not practical for elderly. My HIIT is going up and down the basement stairs ten times a day.

It's probably the most dangerous thing I do all day—staircase disaster.

My Florida neurologist was worried about my falling and told me to walk in the pool thirty minutes three times a week. I did it once. After doing ten minutes, I later realized I had hurt my right hip, which still seems tight at times months later.

Have fun and socialize, and develop playlists of favorite music.

Music

I had a song going through my head that I couldn't remember. I knew it was a Dixie Chicks song. Thus, I asked Alexa to play their top songs. About the sixth song sounded familiar.

I posted some lyrics below. I usually have a difficult time hearing the lyrics, but this time, I listened carefully. I became very emotional when I realized what the song was about.

"Traveling Soldier" by Dixie Chicks.

He was waiting for the bus in his army green
Sat down in a booth in a cafe there
Gave his order to a girl with a bow in her hair
He's a little shy so she gives him a smile
So he said would you mind sittin' down for a while
And talking to me, I'm feeling a little low
She said I'm off in an hour and I know where we can go
So they went down and they sat on the pier
He said I bet you got a boyfriend but I don't care
I got no one to send a letter to
Would you mind if I sent one back here to you
I cried
Never gonna hold the hand of another guy
Too young for him they told her
Waitin' for the love of a travelin' soldier
Our love will never end

In Dr. Daniel Gibbs's book *A Tattoo on My Brain*, on page 147, it states, "For reasons that are still not fully understood, the ability to enjoy, identify and even play music is often preserved even into the latest stages of the disease" (Alzheimer's).

When I go for my mile walk each day, I listen to a playlist on my iPhone. I hear the music directly into my hearing aids. I hear the nuances of the music and the words better than I ever have before hearing aids.

To find new songs, I ask Alexa to play top songs of various artists I like or I recently heard of. I purchased a magazine about Bob Dylan. When I was a senior in high school in 1969, I liked the Beach Boys. In college, I liked the Beatles. Of course, I knew and liked Dylan, but it wasn't till much later I realized how great he was. I listened to cover treatments of his songs and appreciated him more.

This magazine discussed why his top ten songs were so great. This context helped me understand the music so much more.

Final message: If you have early stage AZ, start building your favorite songs into playlists.

CHAPTER 37

Cognitive Reserve with Alzheimer's
August 15, 2021

I was diagnosed with Alzheimer's in December 2017. This month, I was reevaluated by KUMC on my yearly check for my nontreatment research trial number 4. I believe I did well. They don't tell me the result of the three-hour cognitive exam.

MRI report.

Follow-up with my private neurologist.

Am I doing well because I am on the ReCODE protocol, or is it simply that I have a good cognitive reserve?

CHAPTER 38

Fourth MRI For a Nontreatment Trial
August 16, 2021

Today I had my fourth MRI in four years for a scientific trial (nontreatment) that I entered eight months after my diagnosis of Alzheimer's was made in December 2017. Last year, I had QT prolongation on my EKG. Subsequently, my Tau PET scan was cancelled as dictated in the protocol. FDA approved drug used in Tau PET scans.

> While there are FDA approved imaging drugs for amyloid pathology, this is the first drug approved for imaging tau pathology, one of the two neuropathological hallmarks of Alzheimer's disease, and represents a major advance for patients with cognitive impairment being evaluated for the condition.

I was told the trial would start doing the Tau PET scan with me next year. My trial also reaffirmed with me that I was still willing to donate my brain for autopsy. I have never gotten the results of any of my Tau PET scans.

While I remain in mild cognitive impairment, I will continue to do the yearly scans. When I get worse with moderate Alzheimer's, I will get a scan every two years.

It took me a while to get a neurologist to do a MRI on me on February 2017.

My trial mistakenly sent me the results of my first research MRI in August 2018. I was impressed it showed I have normal volume in my hippocampus.

Last month, I asked if I could get another volumetric MRI of the brain where I could see the results. My neurologist said it was not available in private practice. So the MRI I had today, I will never know the results of. My brain autopsy results will be given about one year after my death.

In Dr. Dale Bredesen's patients, he has gotten follow-up hippocampal MRIs in his patients to show they had restored their hippocampus to normal volume after they shrunk by the ReCODE therapy.

Neuraceq 2014 approved to scan for amyloid in brain.

Last year, Tauvid (flortaucipir F18) used to look for Tau was passed by DEA—Tauvid (flortaucipir F18) for intravenous injection, the first drug used to help image a distinctive characteristic of Alzheimer's disease in the brain called tau pathology.

Alzheimer's will become epidemic in the next couple decades. It will probably bankrupt Medicare. Perhaps with early diagnosis, people will do what seems to slow AZ advance. However, the issue must be made a priority by allowing Neuraceq and Tauvid scans covered for the elderly.

CHAPTER 39

On Pluto: First Review
August 17, 2021

I finished reading up to page 163 of *On Pluto* by Greg O'Brien, which I had to stop and start a review.

Part 1 of Review

At this point, I have to be harsh in my review. No question, he is a much better writer than me. I hesitated to buy his book as I thought it might be too dark after I read a dark quote Mr. O'Brien wrote about his present condition.

In 2018, when he revised his book, *On Pluto*, his Alzheimer's was much more advanced than mine is now. I wanted to see what to expect for myself for the future.

One good point he confirms from Gibbs's book *A Tattoo on My Brian* is that I can still do intellectual activities if I have a good cognitive reserve. He says it takes him forty minutes to write what took him five minutes. I suspect he is still trying to maintain high or perfect standards in his writing.

That's his first mistake.

I feel I can be judgmental as I am in year 4 of my Alzheimer's. Don't sacrifice the good for the perfect. No one expects perfection in Alzheimer's.

The second mistake was to not curb his activities earlier in recognition of his Alzheimer's. He writes about many bad outcomes trying to convince himself that he can continue as normal without consequences.

Once I had my diagnosis, I let my medical license lapse. I purchased a much safer Subaru Outback car, and my wife started driving most of the time.

The third mistake was he continued his job.

Living a lie is very stressful. Having a job and then covering up your Alzheimer's lapses would have been impossible for me. For me, a very important part in dealing with my Alzheimer's is avoiding stress. With stress, I get anxious and depressed (see pages 80, 81, and 82).

Fourth mistake was to keep riding a bike (p. 127). After his head injury from a bike ride, he writes, "Little did I know I had released a monster."

The fifth and most severe mistake that affected his family was thinking he could make major decisions about the care of his parents.

He has Alzheimer's, yet when the family comes to the moment of whether to put his mother in a nursing home and the split vote comes down to him making the decision, he decided to keep her in her home with him (p. 126).

"Confusion gave way to chaos. Mom began putting garbage into the trunk of her car."

I got angry at this point. I worked in nursing homes as a geriatric doctor. My wife worked as a nursing home administrator. Family cannot do a good job of taking care of Alzheimer's 24/7. The stress will cause them to abuse the people they are taking care of.

Later, Mr. O'Brien proves my point on page 139 when he yells at his father on his deathbed, "So WHY DON'T YOU TRY NOW TO DIE WITH SOME DIGNITY, DAD, AND TAKE CARE OF MOM ALONG THE WAY!"

"Dr. Robert Harmon saw that my mother was moving from mid s stage Alzheimer's to End Stage, called for family intervention" (p. 136).

The author writes, "Deep into confusion myself and quietly questioning my logic I cast the deciding vote to, Mom and Dad would stay at their home."

Sixth mistake: *Not* sharing his concerns with his wife.

With Alzheimer's, it is essential to share the emotions with your wife.

"I never confided in Mary Catherine [his wife] about this" (p. 140).

CHAPTER 40

On Pluto: Second Review
August 18, 2021

This time I will post what I think Greg O'Brien got right:

1. Exercise

    The author says it recharges his brain. He does a great deal of running. I suspect it's one of the main reasons he is hanging on with moderate severe Alzheimer's. He does seem to pay a price with subsequent body pain. Pain causes distress, and this is not a friend to the AZ brain.

2. Medications (p. 23)

    This is the only AZ book that, at the beginning of the book, discusses the usual medications for AZ.

    *   Aricept.
    *   Namenda.
    *   Trazadone to help him sleep.
    *   Celexa (citalopram), 20 mg.

- An antidepressant for his rage, which considering how bad his rage is, I can't believe he is not on 40 mg, which I take.

3. Socialization

   Mr. O'Brien has a lot of friends that he stays in touch with and gets good support.

4. Hard drive memory palace on office wall (p. 14)

   "They paint word pictures. Everywhere there are historical, FRAMED front page stories and magazine covers."

   My memory palace to remember my family.

   Memory is not what it is cracked out to be.

5. Supplements (p. 193)

   I have only read to page 217 so far. I don't know which specific supplements he takes. The list below is what his Alzheimer's doctor advises:

   - Tru-Niagen
   - Percepta
   - Vegan Omega 3
   - Quercetin
   - Fiscetin
   - TUDCA
   - Ashwagandha
   - Vitamin D3
   - Methyl B12 plus
   - Coenzyme Q (especially if on a statin)
   - Selenium
   - Nordic Natural Probiotic plus prebiotic

6. Religion/Faith

   This is a good strategy when faced with death. Raised as a Roman Catholic, the author draws strength, solace, and some tranquility from his faith.

7. Sleeps seven to eight hours a night
8. Great discipline with memory helpers on his phone and Gmail.
9. Author writes two hours every night.

   I also try to write in my blog and Twitter every day. I feel great gratification when I can write a good thread on Twitter or a good blog. I incorporated my blogs into my last three books on my AZ, which I documented in diary form. I am now working on my year 4 book.

The author and the author of *A Tattoo on My Brian* both taught me about cognitive reserve, which will hopefully allow me to continue my writing even as I enter moderate Alzheimer's.

CHAPTER 41

On Pluto: Third Review

I have read page 341, last page is 364. Time to write the third review of *On Pluto* by Greg O'Brien.

This is a good book.

I was a little critical at first because of his use of stories from other sources to be funny or illustrate his points, most of which I have heard before. Probably I am jealous of all his contacts. He even name-drops people from his childhood in Rye, New York.

This book is long because it is an autobiography. Again, his life is much more interesting than mine. I don't have one-tenth of his friends. I know he is making a context, which is fine.

The chapter that won me over was the one written by his wife, Mary Catherine McGeorge O'Brien, chapter 24, pages 329 to 341.

This chapter is amazing, and I hope my wife will read it.

"Ironically, Alzheimer's now is starting to heal our marriage."

Hopeful words for my wife and I.

In chapter 23, Greg O'Brien puts his investigative reporting skills in action describing how twelve different Alzheimer patients he knows dealt with their Alzheimer's. It is very well-written, with the title "Which One of You Nuts Has Any Guts?"—a quote taken from *One Flew Over the Cuckoo's Nest*, but very apt.

I love his historical references because some of them I was not well acquainted with. Sports references are likewise fun for me and because I heard them for the first time. Popular TV and movie culture references were not so much appreciated as they were very familiar to me, as well as his jokes that I have heard before.

I guess I am being a tough critic. Again, probably jealousy, as he has gotten so much attention.

When I finish reading his book soon, I will write a book review for Amazon. I will say this book has done a great service for me. It is the only book written in the first person that informs me what to expect as I advance from early Alzheimer's to moderate Alzheimer's. The hopeful news is that I will be able to write and talk.

One thing I will do differently: I will take stronger drugs for depression if needed. I am doing well with Citalopram, 40 mg. He only takes 20 mg.

If I had his level of rage, I would definitely take stronger drugs. I know I would not want to put my wife through that, and she would not tolerate it. I would be in a nursing home.

I have more rage than ever, but I have never acted out as he has. I also listen to the people around me telling me what to do. As his wife says, he is an asshole. No humor or jealousy involved.

I gave up my license to practice medicine and decreased my driving. He continues working and puts himself in impossible situations, which cause him great stress. I try to avoid stress. Stress is not good for Alzheimer's.

Distress causes decreased judgment, anxiety, and depression. I will have a cocktail after an argument with my wife to relieve the stress. Ashwagandha has helped me as well. He says he is taking supplements, but he doesn't say which ones other than what Dr. Rudolph Tanzi advises.

CHAPTER 42

Let Me Finish My Damn Sentence!
September 9, 2021

Something I have not seen written anywhere is that people don't allow me to finish my sentences. They anticipate what I am going to say; they are usually wrong.

I have learned not to get angry and start yelling. I am surprised that the other person wants to continue his side of the discussion. I try to point out calmly that because he has not allowed me to finish my side of the discussion, he doesn't even know the point I am trying to make.

I have learned not to get crazy about it.

CHAPTER 43

Review of *The First Survivors of Alzheimer's* by Dr. Dale Bredesen
September 10, 2021

I preordered this new Bredesen book, and it finally arrived yesterday. This is the first book to answer the question I asked in a blog in June 2021: Who are the AZ survivors?

I started the ReCODE protocol after reading about Julie G. First visit to Atma Clinic on October 6, 2020.

With the six survivors discussed in this book and the new AZ drug that seems to be questionable at this point, I feel validated in my decision to start the program at Atma Holistic Clinic in Lawrence, Kansas.

Also after ten months on the program, I am tolerating all the supplements and cost. I also feel better. I did well, I think, on my extensive three-hour yearly cognitive test this week for the nontreatment trial I am in. My fourth MRI result.

Back to the review of *The First Survivors of Alzheimer's: How Patients Recovered Life and Hope in Their Own Words*.

BRIAN SCOTT EDWARDS, MD, FNLA

I loved Daniel Gibbs's book *A Tattoo on My Brain* and Greg O'Brien's book on their personal experience with Alzheimer's. Now Dr. Bredesen's book discusses six of his patients.

His introduction is excellent.

The meat of the book:

- Page 19—Kristen (first patient on ReCODE for nine years)
- Page 45—Deborah (memory improved considerably)
- Page 55—Edward (positive PET scan)
- Page 67—Marcy (chelations)
- Page 87—Sally (IV anti-amyloid medicine made her worse)
- Page 96—Frank (nine years, maintains improvement)
- Page 128—Julie (coauthor of second book, *The End of Alzheimer's Program*)

CHAPTER 44

Supplements Advised by Isaacson and Chris Ochner

Best chapter I have read on supplements for AZ is in *The Alzheimer's Prevention and Treatment Diet* by Richard Isaacson and Christopher Ochner.

The following supplements are advised:

- B vitamins
- Vitamin D3
- Omega-3 fatty acids
- Cocoa powder
- Curcumin
- Resveratrol (I was told by my Atma ReCODE doctor that a couple of glasses of red wine is not enough resveratrol)

They may need an update, as in *The End of Alzheimer's Program* by Dr. Dale Bredesen, they leave out many other options. The ReCODE protocol by Bredesen does include all the above, but Ochner does not advise ginkgo biloba or coenzyme Q.

CHAPTER 45

Return from Three Weeks in Paris During COVID-19

September 20, 2021

Overall, this trip was more challenging to me than prior trips. This time, we had to make certain our COVID-19 test was in time for when we boarded the plane. Suddenly, everyone in Kansas seemed to be testing themselves at the drug stores because of the recent surge. We had a difficult time finding somewhere to be tested. After a couple attempts, we succeeded.

The flights over to France went well, except we were stuck in a long chaotic line in de Gaulle airport to get through customs. People wore masks from all countries, but it was very close quarters.

We entered our Viking cruise, which felt like coming home. The first thing we were required to do was a saliva test. They wanted 2 cc of spit. Took many attempts to fill that much.

By the end of two weeks, I became very accomplished at producing enough after two spits.

Two days after the first test, while on a bus tour, six people were pulled off our bus because two in their party tested positive for the virus. Remember, everyone on the cruise had proof of full COVID-19 vaccination.

On the next separate cruise, no one tested positive the whole week. We were worried because those people were taken off our bus. Of course, we were required to wear our masks on the bus, and it was effective. We were concerned after the close concentration of mixed people at de Gaulle, even though all those people had to be vaccinated. The delta variant can be carried by everyone and spread to the vaccinated, but we did well wearing masks.

We had great weather in the three weeks we were in South France. The two Viking cruises were in the wine country. I was surprised to learn that most of the great Bordeaux wines are blended with four types of grapes. The Beaujolais wine I get in America is weak, and I never found one I liked. In the region where it is grown, it's very good. Beaujolais is generally made of the Gamey grape, which has a thin skin and is low in tannins.

Between Viking cruises, we did a three-day layover at Carcassonne. It has a tremendous castle at the top of the hill. We had a nice efficiency rental at the base of the hill. My friend and I climbed up. It was clearly too difficult a walk for our wives.

We got to the top slowly because I can't walk as well as I used to, and my balance is bad on the uneven cobblestones due to my Alzheimer's.

At the top are some hotels, which I advise because they provide transportation up the till. Great restaurants are up there also.

Going downhill was very treacherous for me. I have festinating when I go downhill. I know how to avoid it by keeping my toes pointing out, landing on my heels, and keeping my head back. It's difficult to keep my head up and back while I have to look where to step. I made it, but I did not go back the next day with my friend.

The only mishap on the cruise was on the second night at the bar. I have the drinking package, which is great as I try everything. I have tried to keep it under control by drinking a glass of water between cocktails. It didn't work out as I had planned.

I got up off the barstool and dropped like a pile of rocks. I hadn't even tried to take the first step.

I didn't hit my head. God watches over drunks and children.

In two seconds, three staff members picked me up and took me to my room, where my wife was sleeping. Surprise!

Last year, just before COVID-19 was bad, we had a party with my family, and I got very drunk. I fell into my bedroom and hit my head. Later, I found out I had a subdural. I am on Xarelto, a blood thinner. I stopped drinking alcohol for two weeks. I finally started drinking again and have tried to not overdo it, except for this recent cruise. I usually have a Manhattan (3 oz. alcohol) after lunch and later with dinner. After that, I have two glasses of wine (total 2 oz. alcohol). That is probably a low amount that I aim for.

Most authorities say this is a high amount of alcohol, especially for someone with Alzheimer's. Many Alzheimer's specialists allow a couple of glasses wine a week. There are studies that show high alcohol shrinks the hypothalamus. I have had two volumetric MRIs over the last four years, and my hypothalamus has not shrunk.

CHAPTER 46

Final Advice for Everyone
September 12, 2021

The subtitle for this book is "True Grit and Fortitude" required. I have tried to simplify what I think is the easiest path, but it still requires a great deal of effort. I have been able to take twenty pills a day even during my three weeks in France last month.

A. The most essential things to do during your lifetime

1. Control blood pressure.
2. Lower cholesterol (LDLc) to less than 100.
3. Check for prediabetes every year.
4. If you are prediabetic, go on the Atkins diet or low carb, high fat diet to get into nutritional ketoacidosis.
5. Walk at least twenty minutes a day.
6. Do weight lifting three days a week.
7. Check your genetic status for Alzheimer's.
8. Sex is good exercise, and Viagra-type drugs help brain blood flow

Easy supplements to take:

- Dark chocolate 90 percent block each morning melted with coffee (flavonoids)
- Drink one glass of red wine a day
- Vitamin D, 2,000 IU a day
- Lovaza (generic available), two capsules a day—take after a fatty meal
- Probiotic

B. Lose weight and maintain the weight loss with Ozempic shot

- C-Socialization
- Treat any suggestion of depression

Signs of depression:

- Lack of energy
- Apathy

C. Get a lab from a doctor each year

- Check vitamin D level
- Lipid panel
- Usual chemistry and Hgb

D. Advice from nutritional therapist at Atma Holistic Clinic

1. I have replaced my diet Powerade with water. I drink 60 oz. of water a day.
2. Add spinach to my eggs in the morning. Eggs are good for choline.
3. Add color to my diet such as berries and sweet peppers.
4. She allows me one Manhattan cocktail each day as an anchor for me.

5. She wants me to eat liver, but I can't stand the taste of it.
6. Start learning a language each day with Duolingo.
7. learn to play an instrument.
8. Make more playlists of music to listen to.

CHAPTER 47

Decision to End Long Driving Trips
October 11, 2021

My wife and I drove from Topeka to Asheville. She does almost all the driving. It is a sixteen-hour drive.

On the first leg to Paduka, I only drove an hour on the highway to give her some rest. She has some trouble in cities and especially with merging in heavy traffic. She also doesn't like it when I speak up about when to turn and gets confused, so she has asked me to not say anything unless it is to avert an accident. If we take a wrong turn, we will just turn back.

She is beginning to have some road rage with foul language. This distresses me. The stress causes me anxiety and depression.

The second leg of the trip, she drove the whole way to Asheville. Of course, after driving for eight hours, she got very tired. It may not be reasonable for me to expect better behavior from her.

We had a wonderful room on the twelfth floor of the Cambria Hotel in downtown Asheville. The view of the mountains was wonderful. Not much color in the leaves yet. Not much sun, but the clouds of fog covering the hills was spectacular from our corner room with wraparound windows. The hotel required everyone in the hotel to wear masks except when eating or drinking. The location was perfect for walking to all the interesting restaurants and stores. The museum was pleasant but did not contain much. The stellar attraction was the Biltmore Manor. The restaurants were good with an emphasis on farm-to-table food. They also tried to make traditional dishes a little different. For a foodie, this might be very interesting.

Four of our friends planned all this in honor of my seventieth birthday coming up in December. They did a great job with the planning. I have known the two couples since my days growing up in Brooklyn, New York.

After a great week, we started our trip home. We had a reservation in Branson (music capital of the world), but I asked Ginger if we could go home. Her friends had cancelled going with us, and while I love music more than ever, I missed my home base, where I have a routine I love.

I maintained my morning fasts and avoided desserts. I was able to continue my important prescribed medications but found it difficult to continue my other ten supplements.

My main reason was I wanted to cut short our road trip due to the stress of Ginger's driving.

Sure enough, right out of the gate on the trip home, Ginger had a major rage meltdown. She said she felt rushed, which surprised me because we got out on time after waking up early. Our major mistake was to not check the side mirrors after the parking attendants handed the keys over to us. Ginger didn't realize it until she tried to merge on the main highway. She had to stop at the end of the merging lane, and to add insult to injury, the car she thought was not allowing her to merge in honked at her. Ginger melted down in a burst of profanities. We finally pulled over and got the mirrors working after she kept saying with anguish the mirrors were broken.

I was determined we would never take another long driving trip without another good driver. Just too much stress for me.

Personal History Before Alzheimer's Diagnosis

For those fans who have enjoyed the first three years of my life with Alzheimer's, I thought I would share my biography before I was diagnosed with AZ.

My earliest memories come from Japan while my father served in the air force. I remember the smell of sweet manure as we drove through small villages.

We moved to a base in Northern Maine, where the first day my brothers and I rode a sled down the hill behind our house off a ballistic early warning radar base. I was seated in the front of the toboggan, and the snow was flying in my face. What great fun!

Caswell was very rural and not far from Loring Air Force Base. I learned to read with Dick and Jane books in a two-room schoolhouse that had students from first to eighth grades. School was let out when potatoes were harvested. I wanted to pick potatoes, but my Dad would not let me.

School began in earnest when we moved back to where I was born in Brooklyn, New York. My education began in earnest and not just in school.

First day after moving into a three-story apartment building on the corner of Nostrand and Avenue D above a pharmacy, my brother, two years older than me, walked to the asphalt park outside of Public School 89. It was a shock to see a block-long park full of kids of all ages playing all sorts of games and somehow not getting in each other's way. Softball, stick ball against the wall. It had a small fenced-off dirt area where games by younger kids like me were played. It was paradise, but they used words I never heard before on the air force bases. I asked my brother what *fuck* meant. Some boys used it constantly. He wouldn't tell me what it meant.

My grammar school had great teachers and a swimming pool. I learned how to rescue drawing people and how to float by taking my pants off, tying the bottom of the legs, and then flipping over the pants to capture the air in the legs and float with it. Never had to use this trick.

My oldest brother was five years older than me. He would take me to the Museum of Natural History, the Museum of Modern Art, the Metropolitan Museum of Art, and the Frick Collection. He was my best and earliest teacher of science and exploring New York City. He taught me the components of an atom. He drew the nucleus with protons and neutrons and the electrons circling around it. I was fascinated.

I met my Bruce on the IRT subway going to Manhattan. We were both going to Stuyvesant High School. He was a junior, and I was a sophomore. We had recognized each other from playing against each other in a church basketball league. That was September 1967.

Now, fifty-four years later, we are still best friends. We both went to Brooklyn College.

Chris was my older brother's friend from Midwood High School. They were in the same year, and he also played for a rival church team. Chris is a unique friend of the family. My oldest brother helped him get a job at Kings County Hospital. Turned out that Chris had a real aptitude for lab work. It became his life-long career, and he became very successful. Chris also became good friends with my parents and stayed in our basement for different periods.

I am still good friends with Chris. Because of his medical background, he was my first friend that I told about my Alzheimer's diagnosis back in 2018 on a Hawaii trip.

FINAL WORD

I have written this series of yearly books to document my experience with Alzheimer's in the first person to show people what they might expect when they first get the diagnosis.

My diagnosis was made in December 2017. Despite being board certified in geriatric medicine, I had no idea what my prognosis was.

It is four years later. I am amazed at how well I have done.

This last year, we were in COVID-19 shutdown. It caused me to refocus my goal from just having fun with travel to trying another alternative path to treatment: Dr. Dale Bredensen's ReCODE protocol from his book *The End of Alzheimer's Program*. Is that what made a difference? Perhaps. I think my aggressive treatment of cholesterol and blood pressure is the most important reason I have not fallen off a cliff, which often causes sudden deterioration in Alzheimer's patients.

My fifth year book will be titled "Avoiding Falling Off Cliffs with Alzheimer's."

I still drive locally. On October 11, 2021, I drove myself about a mile to the grocery store and did the post-Asheville shopping. I know the store well, and as I go up and down the aisles, I know what to buy. I have a backup list in my pocket, but I really don't need it.

I am presently rereading Bernard Cornwall's series about Richard Sharpe. I sometimes remember some poignant sections, but mostly it is as if it is a new read.

Socially, I do better than when I was a young man. Now on cruises, I say hello to almost everyone and strike up a conversation.

On the Asheville trip in October, I had a great time talking science with Chris and politics with Chris and Bruce.

I feel very good about myself. I sleep well with magnesium threonate, melatonin, and Ashwagandha. I rarely have any pain. My depression is controlled with Citalopram 40 mg a day. I believe my anxiety from Alzheimer's is better with Ashwagandha twice a day. I also will pace to help anxiety sometimes.

My self-esteem is high due to the publishing of my books.

Taking all the medications and supplements requires commitment. This is where true grit and fortitude are required. I would never tell anyone this is the cure to Alzheimer's. We don't even know what causes Alzheimer's, let alone how to cure it. This is why my early books before COVID-19 advised patients to just have fun. With COVID-19, I was able to increase my program to include new supplements and to adhere to a regular routine. This routine adds to my contentment.

Cancer patients have been told they need a better attitude for recovery. This is nonsense. Of course, if they are truly depressed, they should take antidepressants. I don't feel sorry for myself with the diagnosis of Alzheimer's. Two friends who were extremely strong physically came down with cancer this year. The eighty-year-old man died this month after astounding Marines at a fair as to the number of pull-ups he could do. I thought he would make it to one hundred years old. My other friend liked to do manual labor, especially building things. He is my age, and to my shock, he has been diagnosed with cancer. Both these men always seem to be upbeat. I write about the need for true grit and fortitude. However, if I had a painful cancer, I would run to palliative care.

We did well on our recent two Vikings cruises in France. No meltdowns and no major mistakes. Ginger was challenged when she was informed that a leg of our flight home was cancelled. British Airway informed us of the cancellation of the first leg of our flight at 1:00 a.m., and there were no other flights leaving Lyon. Ginger was up all night trying to find another flight home. I slept while she worked. I used to do many of the reservations, but she does them all now. She was able to get home at the same time as the prior flight was to get us there. We spent one more night near the airport and flew to Madrid. Very nice.

Lightning Source UK Ltd.
Milton Keynes UK
UKHW010100120122
396998UK00008B/354/J